DEATH

INTERRUPTED BY

LOVE

DEATH

INTERRUPTED BY

LOVE

A True Story

Written by
Anessa L. Haney

To order additional copies of this book, contact:
Xlibris Corporation
1-888-795-4274
www.Xlibris.com
Orders@Xlibris.com
67966

CONTENTS

Dedicated to
~Serena~Marisa~Derrek & Jade

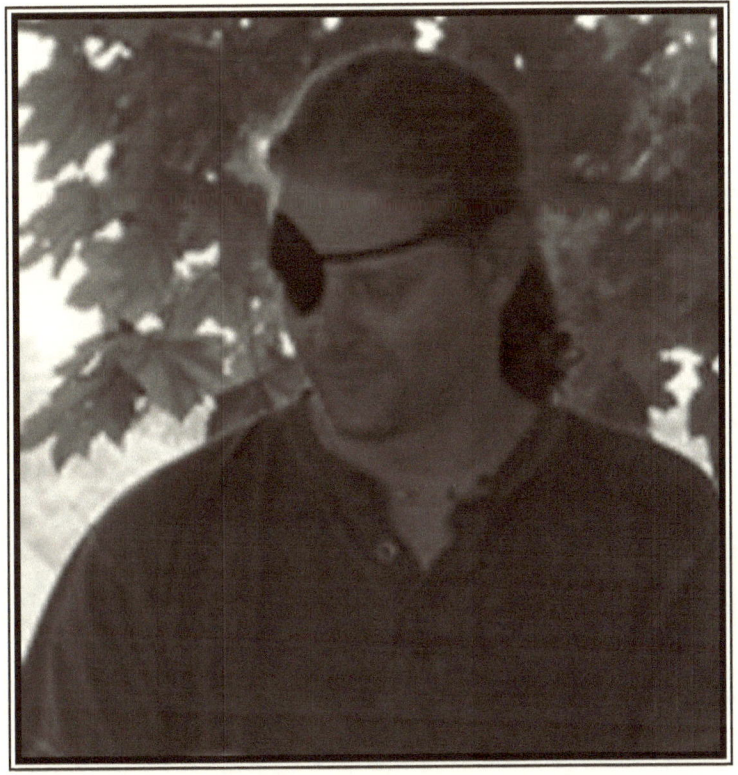

"Edward John Haney"

A special thank you to~

Noah Smith
Raina
Carl Lake
Butch & Julie
Sherry Curran
Sue McElaney
Melinda Santoro Kipp Gardiner
&
The Dream Foundation

Dear Serena,

You have been my *inspiration*, my *drive*, my *hope*, my *cause*, my *ambition*, my *love* and my very *reason for living*. You are a genuine gift from God and you are a beautiful and a mighty asset to mankind.

Remember to love yourself, always, and keep your heart light and open. You have suffered but you have survived. Sweet Serena you are strong and you are my **true joy**.

I love you and I need you to know; Mom and Dad will always love you—No matter how far away we may seem . . . .

Love,
Mommy

SERENA

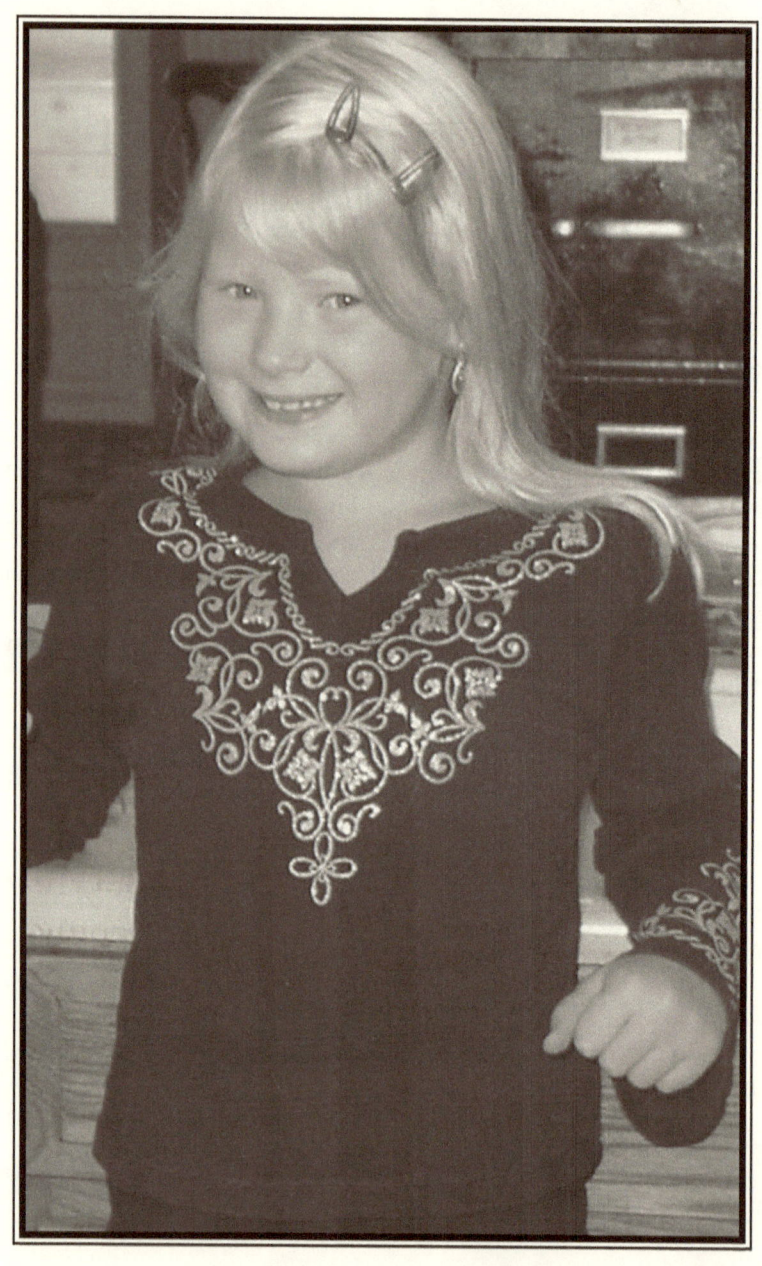

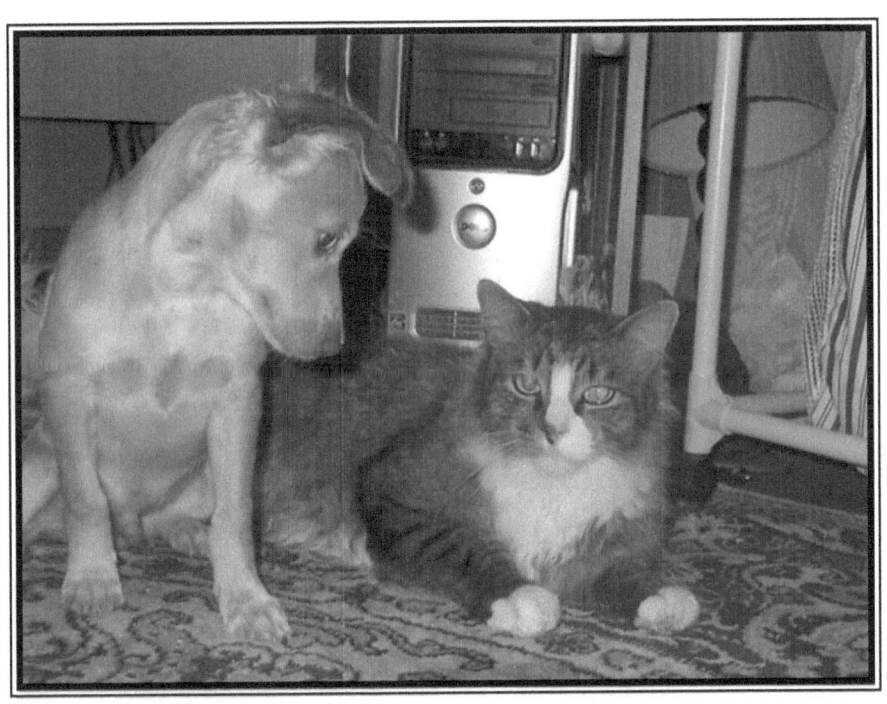

SONNY & SAGWA

Sagwa was Eddie's "prescription cat" He actually had a doctor's note which stated that Eddie needed his cat for therapy-

Sonny was Serena's and my therapy dog after Eddie died, but sadly Sonny was killed by a mail truck.

No Response

"I'm so sad Serena that I have to tell you this; Daddy isn't feeling good honey, so we have to take him to the hospital when we get back from the Magic Kingdom; that means we can't stay too long. We'll take some pictures together and we'll ride some rides and we'll even get some candy and souvenirs, but after that we have to come back and bring Daddy to a doctor."

Ed was getting headaches; they were coming and going and he seemed to have an ear infection because there was clear liquid slowly draining from his right ear. I called one of Eddie's family members, a nurse; she said "it's probably allergies"; I feared it was much worse and truth is I really had no idea what was going on with his ear; I just wasn't comfortable with his condition.

His speech was much more slurred than usual; it was hard to understand him. The tumor started to complicate his speech over the past couple of months, but I had never heard him slur this much; the last time he slurred badly was the day I called his doctor and told him *I* thought the tumor was growing, in the summer of 2006. So, when his speech was slurred in 2007 at the start of our family vacation I grew very worried.

To kill his pain he asked me to pick him up some Advil. And he started taking four milligrams of steroids; two milligrams more than usual. His doctor gave him the go ahead back in Connecticut to take the steroids as needed; the problem this time was that we weren't aware that he was displaying signs of an impending stroke.

Earlier that morning while Serena and I were eating breakfast at the hotel restaurant I asked our waitress for directions to the nearest hospital and I wrote them on a napkin. We had just arrived in Florida two days before and it was only three weeks earlier that The Dream Foundation answered a dying wish for Eddie; a wish to make sure that before he died, Serena be given a trip to Disney; he wanted to give his baby something special because he loved her so much; she was daddy's little girl for sure.

More than to show her that he loved her, I believe it was his way of saying he was sorry for dying and leaving her without him to protect her. I knew it was my duty to ensure that Ed's "wish" for Serena came true; we both knew that if we ended up in the hospital before the trip to the Magic Kingdom, that the whole trip would have been a failure for our baby girl. We made the choice to give our daughter the chance to go to Disney; if we ended up at the hospital first, Serena wouldn't have had any good memories of Disney; all she would have remembered about her trip to Florida would have been traumatic.

After breakfast we walked back to our room; I sat down next to my husband and said "Babe, when we get back you must go to the hospital because I'm worried about you honey. I'll take Serena to Disney but we won't be gone long. I'll be back in three hours." "Yes, you better take that baby! This is for her Nessa, for her! Go and have fun for me, I love you." Sometimes I think that he held out on dying until he knew Serena was in a happier place; a "magical" place.

We gathered up our purses and for a moment we snuggled up to Eddie and kissed him good-bye. But leaving him was extremely hard to do because I was worried that he was going to die from some complication surrounding his tumor; the journey to Disney on that day, to me, was not a journey of fun but one of duty.

I was in such a rush to get through as much of the Magic Kingdom as we could. I wanted Serena to see everything in just three hours; obviously not a likely goal but I was feeling so guilty that she was going to miss out on her dream vacation.

I took some photos of Serena for her to take back to Connecticut to show her second grade classmates; but my worries were deep, so there was no way I could enjoy myself. I put on a fake smile for my daughter's sake; inside I was so anxious and I couldn't stop thinking about my husband and I was scared to death that **"today's the day"** and my overwhelming instincts told me to get ready for the worst; one could say that I was already mentally prepared to find him at the hotel either dead or near it.

I waited until we were through with the Magic Kingdom before I told Serena my fears. She was always well informed about her father's condition because I felt if she had any voids of information she wouldn't be able to grow into a healthy adult. And please believe me when I say this, I wish I could have spared her the reality of her father's imminent death but I just couldn't because we were all in it together; by no means is cancer a personal disease.

I had to tell her my fears so I said "Serena, I am telling you this not to scare you but to prepare you sweetheart because I just need you to be ready; when we get back to the hotel I need you to be brave because I think in my heart that there is a chance Daddy could be dying".

Nearly three hours after we had left him; we pulled into our assigned parking spot at our Resort Hotel in FL. I helped Serena out of the car and I took her hand and we walked into the room; the curtains were closed and the room was dark. I turned on the lights and I said "Hi honey, we're back". I saw Eddie sleeping in the bed and I could hear him snoring very loudly so I walked over to his side of the bed and I pulled the blanket off of him.

His eyes were wide open so I thought he was awake looking at me when I said his name; I didn't get any reaction from him. I said "Ed, Ed?" But still, there was no movement, not even a blink; instantly, I was panicked! From the corner of my eye, I noticed some ice water in a cup on his end table. I dipped my fingers in it and I started to flick the cold water in his face so I could get some sort of reaction; after three tries he still didn't respond.

Meanwhile, Serena was watching me frantically try to wake her father with the ice water, with no luck. When that didn't work I ran over to the other side of the king size bed and I picked up the phone and called 911. As I was on the phone with dispatch, I could see Serena at Ed's side of the bed; she was copying me and splashing her daddy with water to wake him. *It was so painful to watch.*

In what seemed only seconds, the fire and emergency rescue arrived to the first, worst, scene of my life. One of the rescue crew members escorted Serena out of the room and stayed with her on the side walk. I was answering all of the questions about Ed's health. I explained that he had a tumor on his brainstem and that he was acting unusual for the past 24 hours.

On the inside I was so scared and I felt so much guilt for leaving him that morning! No one could wake Eddie. The rescue workers tried for about ten minutes but still they couldn't; he was put up on a stretcher and placed in an ambulance and then he was transported to "Celebrity" (*the name has been changed—to avoid some controversy*) Hospital in Florida. I gathered up my baby and we got in the car and followed the ambulance to the hospital.

DIAGNOSIS

2002. Eddie was an electrician, working for a great company; he loved his job building gas stations. He was looking fine; his body was in great condition; he was tan and muscular and even his hair was, as he would say in his Elvis voice, "perfect".

Although Eddie was apparently healthy on the surface, he started to complain that while he was at work he would have double vision while he was climbing ladders, and he was getting dizzy because his balance was off too. He told me that his partner John had to drive the company truck home each day while he would sleep; his lethargic nature was most alarming to him.

In 2002 Serena and I had great State health insurance but Eddie had none. Well, it was around that time that I started to get recognized in my community for some projects that I spearheaded; I had become active in my *Putnam, Connecticut* community. And with my new report, I was soon recognized by the North East Department of Health's director, Pat.

Pat approached me one day and asked if I would like to participate in a community based outreach program. One of my responsibilities was to take a college course; it was a state grant, at Three Rivers Community College. In that class I learned about the State "Husky" program, health insurance for children and families. It was during that class that I realized that Eddie was eligible for the same great benefits Serena and I had.

With all the dizziness and balance issues, I moved quickly to obtain some insurance for my husband. I completed all of the necessary forms and I sent out Eddie's application for health insurance. And within only a week or so we heard back from a State social worker. She told us Eddie was insured under the State program.

A couple of days later, on September 09, 2002; I asked Eddie to take the day off from work and go to the Day Kimball Hospital ER. Even though he hated to call out of work, he agreed to go.

At the ER Eddie explained, to the ER doctor, what was going on with his health; he told him about the dizziness, the double vision and the lethargy. And after listening to Eddie, the doctor concluded that he was 99.9% sure that Ed had Lyme disease. But just to be sure, the doctor ordered up an M.R.I.

About an hour or so later the doctor returned with the devastating results of the M.R.I; the results were horrifying; Eddie had a large tumor sitting on his brainstem. I was shocked and instantly frightened by the unknown. Literally, all I could say was "shit!" It was so surreal to me. Our lives were full of so much potential and joy, then WHAM!!!

The ER Dr. arranged for an ambulance to transport Eddie to a well known and respected hospital in Connecticut. He said Eddie needed to be looked at by a neurologist because his condition was too rare and sensitive for the hospital he was at to handle. So we called our parents to let them know what was going on; we needed their support. And about an hour later both of our parents were at the hospital.

My parents came to take Serena home with them; Serena was less than two years old at the time. After they took Serena, I prepared myself for the trip to The hospital; I moved my Dodge Ram van and parked it in a place it could stay for a couple of days. Then Eddie and I left in the ambulance together.

So, there we were in the ambulance together getting ready to embark on the most miserable journey two lovers could ever take together, the journey of death.

Two hours later, we arrived at The hospital and we were escorted to a private room; The hospital was always accommodating to me throughout the next *four* years. The private room gave us the chance to open up right away; we were able to talk and cry together. Actually, only I cried, he never cried about it, not until 2006.

Over the next two days we talked about lots of things; everything from our fears to our love for one another. And finally, on September 11, 2002 Eddie was scheduled for a brain biopsy; we were anxious to find out if his tumor was malignant or benign. I can remember that I was amazed at how calm he was; unlike me. I was crying and clinging tightly to him when the anesthesiologist arrived to take him to the O.R. I told him I loved him deeply and kissed him, and then she rolled him off through the double doors of the O.R.

I was all alone with no family and no friends to sit by my side as I cried and cried and cried. I was mostly afraid that Eddie wouldn't make it out of his surgery alive. I just didn't know what to think or how to feel; all I could do was cry my eyes out and very anxiously wait for him to come out of his surgery.

There was no sitting still for me; I made several stops to the receptionist's desk to check my husband's status. At that time I was a rookie to the medical world, unlike today. Then, I barely understood the word biopsy, let alone malignant and benign. So I simply did not know what to expect from this thing called "biopsy". I just kept thinking that brain surgery would leave Eddie like a vegetable or something; I was totally ignorant about tumors and brain surgery.

At one point I started to cry publicly so much that I had to find refuge in a more private place, so that I could really let go of my emotions. I found a private stairwell and I cried loudly and like a crazy lady I started to sing "Thank you for being a friend" from the TV show "The Golden Girls". I was insane with despair.

After two procedures, the doctor used the wrong tool the first time; Eddie was finally in my line of vision again. I first noticed him while he was lying on a hospital bed being pushed out of an elevator by a nurse. He had his hand up in the air, it seemed involuntary, and shook it briefly before it dropped to the side of his stretcher. Wrapped around his head was a white cloth with blood leaking through the material; he looked just like a wounded soldier who had been through a round of vicious battle.

When Eddie was settled in his room, together we spoke to his surgeon. He told us that the tumor was considered to be benign, not cancerous, but he ensured us that Eddie's condition was severe. He told us that because of the threatening position of the tumor; it would be in the "cancer category", but it would technically be considered non-cancerous. It was the type of tumor that could never be operated on due to its location; the tumor was brain matter that had turned into a tumor growth on his brainstem; the tumor was a threat because of its location and *experimental* chemotherapy and radiation were the only possible chances for decreasing the size of the tumor.

Eddie went through a variety of medications, including chemotherapy, radiation and steroids. At one point the radiation seemed to help stop the tumor growth, but in 2006, several smaller tumors started to branch off of the first tumor.

Eddie's neurologist didn't start referring to Eddie's condition as "cancer" until the tumors started to grow at an alarming rate. Although the tumors were benign, they were in such a dangerous place, which made them just as deadly as a malignant tumor; his doctors were sure they would kill him someday.

ER

At the ER Eddie was still totally out of it, with a fever of 104. I stopped a nurse and pointed out that he had some clear fluid draining from his right ear. Now, I being a paranoid person; I thought that his tumor was getting bigger and it was leaking from his ear. And I know it sounds crazy, but I was just in a place in my mind where all I could think of was the absolute worst.

I was extremely uptight, especially because of the fact that we were so far from home. It was all up to me to handle everything and everyone; it was bad enough that his family thought it was wrong that I brought him to Florida.

A nurse brought Serena a tray of food. She was sitting in a chair next to her father's bed. She was drawing, as she so frequently would, for her therapy I'm sure. She reached out and grabbed a hold of the tray while she pushed her crayons and paper aside. She was hungry, tired and stressed out from all of the commotion at the hotel and now she was stuck at a hospital.

She was eating her food when the neurologist walked in and introduced himself to me. He told me that he was concerned that the fluid draining from Ed's ear was possibly meningitis and that if he didn't place a ventricular tap, in my husband's head, to drain the excess fluid from his brain, he would soon die. So he asked me for permission to move forward with the procedures. In addition to the drain, he put Eddie on life support because he claimed that Ed would only live for maybe two hours breathing on his own.

Sadly, before I had a chance to say anything to the doctor, in response to his question, Serena stopped eating her food, and she walked over to the doctor and me. She wedged herself between us and she looked up at me and said "No Mommy, don't let them put those tubes in him, let him go to Paradise because you know what the Bible tells you." It was so painful for me to hear my baby, his baby, say "let him go".

Moments before I told the doctor to put him on life support I had spoken to his mother over the phone and she told me that if the doctors needed to do anything "technical" that I should resist being a "hero" and "let him go". But there was no way I was willing to let him go without a fight! It was my duty as his wife to protect him and do what ever I could to save him

Duty is a strong part of my nature, so it was easy for me to speak for my husband and honor his wishes. Besides, I can recall having car problems in the past but I never threw away my car; I just had it fixed, and I thought he could be fixed too!

The procedures began around 3:40 pm. After the surgery started I took Serena and began the tedious course of walking circles around the hospital to kill time. We quickly discovered that "Celebrity" was a very beautiful place; so clean and very spiritual in nature. And it was apparent to see, that the medical staff did not wear scrubs. The doctors, down to the cleaning crew, all wore khaki pants and polo shirts. It was the mission of the hospital to make their patients feel like they were number one. The scrubs would have taken away from the personal feel they were trying to achieve.

There was a large chapel and many large paintings with images of Jesus Christ. It was a very peaceful place. But unfortunately even with all that beauty and serenity, the fact remained that it would soon become a place, for Eddie, of suffering.

My best friend Naomi was supposed to come see Eddie, me and Serena at our hotel that day. She planned on arriving, from Miami, around 5 pm, so I gave her a call to let her know what happened and where she could find us. She was near by when I called her, maybe an hour or so away; it was about that long until the neurologist reported to me that Ed was stable enough to move to the ICU.

In what seemed like seconds after he told me this, Naomi pushed through the double doors of the ER. It was a miracle for Serena and I that she had arrived. I couldn't believe that she was there for us in our darkest time! I hadn't seen her for a couple of years and now here she was, just in time!

CASINO

We met in the spring of 1997 at a popular casino in Connecticut; at that time, I was a sweet and flirtatious nineteen year old girl, and he was a handsome, charming, divorced, twenty-nine year old, father of three.

I simply couldn't avoid his stares as he passed me by each morning on the Rain Maker concourse. Every morning at eight am I would be busy sucking up "dust bunnies" which lurked under every bench, around every trash can, in every corner, and especially under the retail carts. On one particular morning I was going about my normal dust bunny sucking when my cord got tangled up. Instantly, I was frustrated because it was nearly the end of my shift and I didn't have time for that kind of delay. But I was forced to stop what I was doing, despite my woes.

I unstrapped the dust buster from my back and I started to try to unravel the cord but to further add to my aggravation it was tangled pretty badly. In the midst of my frustration, Eddie walked by; he obviously noticed that I was having a problem because he stopped and said "can I help you unravel your cord Miss?" And in my desperation I answered with "thanks, yeah, that would be great." When he was bent down I saw he was a slot technician and his name tag said "Eddie"; I thought, "at least I know his name." He succeeded in the task at hand and I thanked him and in his extremely charming voice he said, "You're welcome Miss" then he walked off.

I felt like a servant girl straight out of a fairytale who had just been rescued by her future prince.

My position at the casino was something like the, second to the last, worst job to have at the casino; It was truly considered, by some people, to be the bottom of the barrel job at the casino, so it was easy to feel like Cinderella.

And I was definitely the best looking person in my department; not to seem conceited or anything, but it was true.

Besides, it wasn't exactly my fault that I ended up in that department; it was my friend Steve who called me one day to let me know that the Casino was hiring for the Department of Interior. Well, I thought it sounded great; I had no clue what it stood for, so like an ambitious ass, I signed up for duty!

On my first night on the job I did my hair and make up perfect! I was ready to go! And when I reported to the D.O.I department I was anxious to see what I would be doing. My new supervisor walked up to me and introduced himself and then he handed me a pan and broom, then he directed me to where I needed to start sweeping and cleaning the casino floor. He also instructed me to pluck, with my fingers, the cigarette butts from the huge ash trays that filled the place.

I did find a crumbled up twenty dollar bill in an ash tray which was cool. But even with my new found fortune it wasn't the kind of work that I expected; one of the worst parts of that job was when I had to wear a vacuum cleaner that looked like a back pack straight out of Ghost Busters the movie.

I had to strap this thing on my back and head out in public and vacuum every dust bunny in sight! Well I was very vain at that age so wearing that back pack was like walking around with a huge pimple on my forehead; it just didn't help my vanity that every morning around eight am three very flirtatious slot technicians would walk down the concourse right through my work area while I had the pack strapped on my back.

The guy in the middle would always be checking me out and chewing on his tooth pick; looking at me like he was going to catch me looking at him. I tried really hard to act like I didn't see him; besides, I wasn't in the mood to get hit on when I was sucking up cigarette butts and toenails left behind by the dirty and barefooted gamblers.

Our paths crossed again; we were both on our breaks when he was standing in line at the soda machine. When I saw him I got excited but I didn't want it to show. I tucked in my name tag so he couldn't know my name; I still don't know why. I was a bit shy when I went up to have my turn at the soda machine. When he saw me, he had a sweet smile on his face; he asked me what my name was and I said "Anessa". "Anessa, ooh I like that." And off he went.

Of course after a few "chance" encounters we started to date and we fell in love. We dated for about two years before we got married in the spring of 1999.

Two weeks after Eddie and I were married in Norwich, Connecticut, we moved to Boulder City, Nevada; we had an awesome time together on our first cross country road trip.

We loved Boulder City because it was such a beautiful town; we always called it our post card town. It was so quaint and romantic. Each night Eddie and I would go for walks together in the Nevada night and we would get ice-cream at the local ice-cream parlor. We would take our time as we walked hand in hand eating our ice creams. It was so romantic and I captured each and every moment I spent alone in the desert with my husband.

We both had great jobs and life was treating us like never before; he was working as slot tech in Las Vegas and I was an office manager for a coffee company.

Although Eddie and I were enjoying life out West, it was less enjoyable for his children back East; they were missing their father and he was missing them too. He felt compelled to go back to the East Coast so he could be closer to them.

On our journey back to Connecticut we stopped at Eddie's brother's home in Georgia. We stayed there for about two weeks. While we were there, on April 23rd 2000 we celebrated our first year wedding anniversary; together we lit our wedding candles and then Eddie lovingly embraced me and told me he was ready to be a father again; it was then that we created our Serena.

We returned home to Connecticut and nine months later Serena was born.

Then one year and nine months after she was born, Eddie was diagnosed with a brain tumor.

Saint John's Wort

It wasn't until December of 2006 that Eddie's condition really started to show its ugly face; he was experiencing extremely high levels of anxiety. He was on steroids to stop the swelling in his brain caused by the tumor. He was stressed about life and he was dealing with malignant issues that weren't even cancer related. It was an all around crisis situation; we were literally living in a hell.

Ed was good at putting on a happy face around others even when he really wasn't happy. But as Eddie's body started to break down, so did his emotions.

When Eddie would go to his neurology appointments and see his doctor, at a well known and respected hospital in Connecticut, he would tell him "You know Doc; I really am pretty much a moody prick". I would agree with him and I pointed out that I thought he was suffering from severe depression; the issue was never taken seriously and it always seemed to me like the doctor and his nurse were just patronizing me. Instead of offering help for Eddie, his doctor told him to just deal with it and realize that it was the steroids; mood swings were taking over Ed's frame of mind; so much that he started to self medicate.

Eddie thought that he could use an herbal remedy to help him deal with his anxiety. I can remember he told his doctor that he doesn't worry about his anxiety anymore because "now I just swallow a handful of St. John's Wort and shut my mouth". He was wrong, it wasn't helping at all because his mannerism was changing and he was becoming highly aggressive . . . Every word had a "fuck" at the end of it. If it was a coffee . . . it was a coffuck . . . a car was a carfuck. Everything coming from his mouth was foul.

In no time at all, a DCF (Department for Children and Families) worker came to our apartment after getting the reports of Ed's aggressive behavior around Serena; just another thorn in the cancer war.

We had all kinds of issues to deal with in our crisis but I never lost sight of the fact that my family needed me to remain focused and strong, so when

I couldn't pin what was going on with my husband it drove me insane with desperation.

Some of Eddie's family members insisted that, "it simply isn't Eddie talking anymore." I just didn't see it the way they did. And Serena was starting to break over Ed's behavior. She would make and throw paper balls at him when he started swearing at me. As soon as he woke up he would say to me "get up bitch! We sleep when we are dead!" "Get up!" I would have no choice but to get up because he just wouldn't stop! It was horrific; I was worried for Serena. The only way we could get away from the torture was to go for a ride in the State forest and stay away as long as we could.

Eddie was acting very aggressive on the day I decided to call 911. I told the dispatcher the situation; that he had a tumor and he needed to be evaluated. I felt so bad for my husband; I mean I can't explain how bad I felt when the ambulance showed up. He was so scared and confused. He was nearing his lasts days of being able to walk so he was very unsteady. He even tried to run and hide from the ambulance by walking down the road but he couldn't make it far. It was so sad to see him trying to escape, so sad. But the police were able to convince him to go to the hospital.

Sadly, it was actually a relief to see him go because it was a break from the abuse. Luckily, on that day, Serena had a birthday party to go to; it was the perfect way to keep her mind off the situation. But not me, I couldn't stop thinking about my poor husband and I was hoping that he was being evaluated and helped.

We returned home three hours later and we walked up to our back door and I looked through the window in the house; I saw Eddie sitting at our kitchen table talking on the phone; I could hear him talking to his sister. I was shocked to see that he was wearing a hospital johnny; I actually thought he escaped from the hospital or something.

When I walked into the house Eddie was instantly irate with me. He said that I had put him in jail (he considered the ride to the hospital jail) and he threatened me with physical pain. He said he wanted a divorce and he wanted nothing to do with me; just acting unlike himself. I was very concerned for him so I reached out to his family for help.

I asked them to separate us for a little while so that we could have some peace but every time his family would come over he would act nice and his mood would change. But I knew he was acting out of character the majority of the time. The day he sat in the kitchen wearing a jonnie, he was dropped off at home by a cab because a doctor sent him home; he said he wasn't a threat to himself. But even though he wasn't a threat to himself, he was to us.

That same night, Eddie was acting out of control; when I picked up the phone to call a friend he threatened to smash the phone; and he did exactly what he had threatened to do, he smashed the phone. So once again I grabbed Serena and we left for yet another ride to nowhere, except out of there.

When we returned home at around two am, he was sleeping. I did not want to wake him because I was afraid that he would go crazy. So, like a soldier, I got down on my belly and I slithered across my living room floor so that I wouldn't get spotted. I was trying to gather up some things and I was picking up the floor of small messes so that when he woke up nothing would spark his rage.

He just wasn't normal and I was losing him. Sometimes it was like he was already dead; he was fading away and to me he sometimes seemed dead and completely disconnected from me. And it absolutely drove me mad with motivation; I needed to figure out what was going on with my man! I never thought it was just the tumor.

The DCF worker suggested that I leave him. When I explained what was happening at our house, she suggested that I leave him. She said he had no excuse to treat others poorly even if he was sick. But I explained to her that it was my goal to make her understand that even though the situation was distressing to me and Serena, that it wasn't a character flaw on Ed's part and that he was only being abusive because something just wasn't normal about him. She believed, like others, that he simply had a bad attitude about death.

Truly, people surrounding us were in denial and they simply could not grasp the depth of Ed's situation. So I had no choice; on Ed's next scheduled chemotherapy appointment, I talked to a social worker and expressed my fears and concerns for Eddie. And right after he was done with his chemotherapy the social worker asked Eddie to come into a small room to talk with her but instantly he became confused and angry over the "interrogation". I understood his anger but I couldn't let him come home for our baby's sake; not until he was properly evaluated.

He started to rage out at me; security was called and Eddie was escorted to the psychiatric unit where he had to spend a few days. I hated the fact that I had to go to that extreme. I never wanted Eddie to feel trapped or beat down; I just loved him too much to let him go unchecked. I needed to find out if he would stay the rage filled person he had become or whether he was going through some unknown medical issue. I just wanted him home, safe, happy and with us.

Mean while, it was only a couple of days before Christmas and DCF was still threatening that Serena would be taken away from me if Ed returned home. So I called the DCF branch and I asked to speak to a DCF supervisor. When we spoke she kept talking down to me and she was really making me mad because she was dictating to me how I was going to live my life and more importantly, she was messing with my child. So, I flat out asked her, "is there a court order or a law prohibiting him from returning home to us?" She said no, so I told her that she had better stop using idol threats toward my family and I told her to back off because it was my goal to get him home, healthy and safe; after all, *he was dying*!!!

On the day the psychiatric doctor released Eddie from the hospital, the chemotherapy nurse called me on the phone. She said Eddie was leaving the hospital but his sister would be picking him up; I picked him up and brought him home on Christmas day 2006. The nurse also said that it hadn't dawned on her, at the time, but when Ed mentioned a couple of times that he was taking St. John's wort to calm his depression, that the combination of chemotherapy and St. John's wort was "the cause for Eddie's psychotic episodes"; according to her, the pharmacist at the hospital's pharmacy told her that the combination of chemotherapy that Eddie was taking, mixed with the St. John's wort, was a toxic combination; he was having a very bad chemical reaction which was causing him to have "psychotic episodes."

After a couple of weeks, Eddie calmed down and we started working on living our lives once more. We started looking to buy a home in Maine and the three of us were living happily without the interruption of rage or DCF! We truly thought things could get better for us.

The Dream Foundation

I never had any desire to visit Florida and the thought of Disney World never really crossed my mind. Unlike most Americans, it was never on my agenda to see Mickey; it wasn't until Eddie bought his sail boat that my whole idea of Florida changed. Eddie always told me he loved Florida and that one day he would sail the three of us there.

As a matter of fact, in the summer of 2006 we were in the process of cleaning, painting and prepping his 25 ft C&C Yacht; we were only a couple of small steps away from being able to purchase a mooring and then finally venture off down the East Coast, toward Florida. We were literally going to pack up our belongings and live our lives on that sailboat.

Sadly, even though Eddie was feeling great and he was under the certain impression that his tumor was no longer growing, and was for the most part no longer a threat; he had one final M.R.I before he finalized his boating dreams. But of course, as fate would have it, the tumor took a sudden course for destruction.

In the summer of 2006 he was re-diagnosed with new, "aggressive" tumors which started to branch off of his first brainstem tumor; we never had the chance to live our dream together. The only thing we got to live was yet another crisis situation.

It wasn't until sometime in February of 2007 that Florida would come up as a topic in our household once again. It came at a time when Eddie was receiving his final round of chemotherapy. It was obvious that his condition had turned terminal; but we remained hopeful.

While Eddie was receiving a round of chemotherapy I went for a walk around the hospital; I couldn't stand being in the chemotherapy unit; the room where the chemo patients received their treatments was wide open and it was fairly large.

There were about twenty red recliners scattered about in the open space. The chairs were the stations that the chemo patients would take during their treatments. I can recall sitting right next to a man who appeared, to me, to be receiving a blood transfusion; in my opinion there was no privacy and no dignity in receiving treatments there.

To add to our aesthetic discomfort, we noticed that there were only a handful of portable tables with wheels; they were food tables, sometimes, and other times they acted as nurses' stations; the nurses would lay a blue chuck on the top, and then line up their supplies, like needles.

The nurses would have to work right out in the open on each individual patient. And I can recall the first treatment Eddie received, the nurse didn't even wear gloves when she drew his blood; of course I pointed it out to her and she so ignorantly stated, "Oh I'm not worried about it." It wasn't her I cared about; it was my husband's health that I was worried for. And I never saw a nurse sanitize the surface after the chuck was removed from the table; they would just push it along to the next person or it was left out for anyone to grab, for food or soda or whatever.

It made me sick to be there; I hated to see the way the place was run. And poor Eddie had to receive his treatments for nearly seven hours at a time; it was an all day event, so I went for walks frequently to get away from the gross energy that I felt when I was at the chemotherapy unit. Often I would walk over to a waiting area that was located on a concourse, hallway, and one floor down from the chemotherapy unit. It was wide open and there were computers to use.

Sometimes I would kill time by researching stuff on the computers; the access was really limited though, so I was lucky that I even found *The Dream Foundation; a beautiful non-profit organization which grants last wishes to terminally ill adults.*

Eddie was never terminally ill, in my mind; it wasn't until he was going through treatments in 2007 that I realized he was truly beginning to cross over the bridge of death; I had several vivid dreams about Eddie before his passing; I knew he was dying because in my dreams he told me so. It was as if the Eddie of my dreams was telling me in advance that the Eddie of the awake, as I knew him, would begin fading away. Sorry, this is probably too deep and too complex for me to put on paper.

Suddenly I found myself on a mission; a mission to give Eddie something bright in his dark time. I wanted Eddie to "live like he was living" and enjoy some good times with Serena and I. We had been through so much together and we all just needed a break from some of the extremely negative energy which surrounded us in Connecticut. So much bad and evil energy, that it took me nearly three years to filter out countless names and incidents; I have tried so hard to eliminate as much controversy as possible. So if my suggestions of a crisis seem vague—it is intended to be.

I wrote down all of the contact information and when we got home I called *The Dream Foundation* and requested all of the papers that I needed to fill out to make a dream request for Eddie. Once I received it I quickly filled it out and sent it back. No more than two weeks later, Eddie was given a response and granted a wish.

Finally, we were going to be freed from our hellish reality, at least for a little while. When Eddie opened up the letter from *The Dream Foundation* it said,

> *"Dear Mr. Haney,*
>
> *You called upon us with a request to manifest a dream for you. We hope to give you back some of the joy and love you have given to your family and friends, as well as others. We are proud to honor you for being an inspiration to others and an extraordinary person. We are pleased to make a dream come true for you. Enclosed, you will find a check in the amount of $1115.00 to assist you with your dream expenses. We hope you have a wonderful time."*

The Dream Foundation didn't just send Eddie their response by mail; they came in person. It was around April 6, 2007 that Eddie and I were most pleasantly surprised by two beautiful angels sent from *The Dream Foundation*. Melissa and Jodi entered our lives bearing gifts of love and compassion; they were sent to us to lift our hearts and help ease some of the pain. They came into our lives at a time when all we had was sadness and despair; Jodi and Melissa were so warm and understanding about our situation. We easily opened up to them and shared our story with them; and in exchange they told us a little about themselves, but mostly they smiled and seemed to admire the love that Eddie and I had for one another.

With them, they had some gifts for Serena and they had all of the trip information for us. It included the check, hotel reservations and of course the magical tickets to Disney. We were amazed at the gifts that were put in front of us; it was surreal in so many ways because at that time we had so many people working against us, but at that moment when Jodi and Melissa were in our home, we felt like there was still hope.

They were going to leave the gifts behind for Serena, but instead they decided that they would go to Serena's school to hand deliver the gifts to her. So I called Serena's school and I asked if it would be ok for *The Dream Foundation* to come to give Serena the gifts. Of course the Principle said yes; the school was so supportive to Serena during her time of struggle with her father's condition. Excitedly, Jodi, Melissa and I drove to the school and surprised an unsuspecting Serena; needless to say, she was very happy and she felt extremely important on that day. It will always stick out in her mind as a good memory, I'm sure.

The next time we heard from *The Dream Foundation* was when Melissa sent us a letter. The letter came a little less than a week after Eddie had passed away. In the letter Melissa asked how we were doing and she gave us her phone number so we could let her know how our trip was. When I called Melissa she told me she had a dream about us and she was worried that something had happened. Well, I informed her of what *did* happen and I gave her the information on how she and Jodie could attend his funeral.

The wake was in Putnam, Connecticut at Gilman and Valde funeral home. Melissa told me they would try to make it; they were not at the wake, but to my surprise they were at the graveyard. When every one of the family members left the graveyard, I was standing next to one of Eddie's best friends, Marcel, and my baby Serena when I turned around and noticed Jodie and Melissa, I couldn't believe they were there! They reminded me of the people from the TV show "Touched by an Angel".

The attendant at the Exeter, Rhode Island Veteran's Memorial graveyard told me it would be just about an hour before Eddie's coffin would be placed in the ground, so we decided to go to a local diner for some lunch together.

What a peaceful thing it was to have their comfort because sadly, at that time I was having some extremely terrible family problems. Serena and I had no family support; the only real support we had came from our dearest friends.

There was a lot of activity going on at the graveyard that day. There was an area that was about the size of an acre which was all dug up; it looked like a construction site before the foundation is laid. There were big bucket trucks that were hauling off dirt and digging grave holes. One of those holes belonged to my husband; I just didn't know which.

Wearing my high heels and black widow's dress, I started to walk toward the work site. The dirt was defiantly ankle deep and I recall the wind was whipping hard around my long hair as I made my way towards the holes.

When I reached a worker I told him who I was looking for; he pointed to a hole. I walked over to it and I looked over the edge. I saw a large cement box deep down in the Earth; the name **Haney** was spray painted on it. And at that moment it was final and it was clear; that hole and that concrete box were my beloved husband's new home.

When I turned back to leave, I saw Serena, Marcel, Jodie and Melissa waiting for me. Thank you Dream Foundation, thank you.

THE COFFINS

The opportunity to purchase the house came after the St. John's wort problem. Things had settled and Eddie was starting to deal with his condition and situation better.

On March 23, 2007, on Eddie's birthday, he was approved for a mortgage loan. In the year 2007 everything that was bad on his credit got deleted or removed because he had gone through his seven years of punishment from the credit bureau. He was eligible to buy a house with his VA home loan program; He was in the Navy during the Gulf War 1988-1992 era. It was a small loan by most standards; $79,000.00 for a beautiful three bedroom home with 2 baths on an acre of land in Milo, Maine which suited our income perfectly.

For two years Eddie and I drove back and forth from Connecticut to Maine to find a new home. We met an agent out in Bar Harbor, Maine by the name of Jeff. He showed us some of the properties we had seen online but we didn't find any that suited us, not even after three trips.

I can remember our last trip; Jeff didn't even recognize Eddie; he was sitting in my car waiting for us to come out of Jeff's office. When Jeff looked out the window and saw a person sitting in my car, he said "Who did you bring along this time?" He didn't realize it was Eddie until I told him that he was waiting in the car. Eddie looked completely different, like a totally changed man, a cancer patient.

Sadly, I can remember Eddie not being able to get out the car; he could barely walk at that point. I remember asking Jeff to help me lift Eddie out of the car so he too could see the house for sale.

But Eddie insisted that he not and that I just look at it and he would take my word for it. It broke my heart that he couldn't get out of the car to look at the house.

A couple of months later when we were in Connecticut, Eddie and I were looking at houses online when we found one we liked in Milo, Maine. We decided that I would journey out to Milo and check it out while he and Serena stayed behind.

I gathered up my stuff and took a short nap with Eddie and Serena; I got up at about midnight and I headed out and I drove until about eight am the next morning.

When I arrived in Milo I met with the agent. When he showed me the house I thought it was perfect for us, and it was just as perfect as the online photo looked; most houses that we checked out from online always turned out to look way worse in person, but not this one, this house was just like it seemed.

After I called Eddie and got his approval to buy it, I spent an hour talking and negotiating with the agent. I made an offer that day and I signed the paper work for the loan. When everything was all set, I called Ed and I headed back to Connecticut.

When I arrived home I was relieved to be with my family and I felt a sense of accomplishment for finding a home that was suitable for Ed's power chair, with lots of space for our family.

At home, I told Eddie all about the Milo house; he would talk about the house with who ever would listen. He would say "you should see it; it's got this huge room here and so much space." He thought the house was perfect and he never even saw the house in person, all he saw was a couple a cheap real estate photos of the place; that's how connected we were to one another.

Even though he never saw the house he knew about it through me. He trusted what I told him and basically he put himself there in his mind. Just like my husband's sailboat, I never had the chance to sail with him but in my mind I believed him that it was going to be beautiful and one of the greatest experiences, so I imagined having that experience with him in my mind. Communicating to Eddie about the house made it real to him which in turn made it real to us.

It had a closing date for May 23rd 2007. We were using the no money down program from the VA. The only out-of-pocket expenses would be the closing costs.

With all of the support and encouragement, Ed was feeling great for a change. Plus, he was off of the drug clonazepam which was prescribed to him after the St. John's wort issue; it was meant to help calm his poor nerves, and it worked because he was beginning to feel alive and happy again.

There it was his 39th birthday, his credit was fixed, he was approved for a house loan and *The Dream Foundation* had just promised him a loving wish; things were looking up for all of us.

One month later, while we were at "Celebrity" Hospital; Ed's brother was there and at that point Eddie was wide awake and he was totally aware of his brother's presence. I liked his presence because he was genuinely concerned and he wasn't there to judge me. I felt comfortable talking with him about our dream of home ownership; I showed his brother the photos of the house and I asked Eddie if he still wanted to get the house and if I should move forward with the agent. He shook his head yes.

Listen, I really believed that my husband was going to live, and that's why I did what I could to keep **our** dream alive. After Eddie gave me the go ahead to call the agent, I did. But I wanted him to know ahead of time what had happened to Eddie. I told him we were still serious about closing but I didn't want to give him false expectations because I realized the volatility of Eddie's situation.

I didn't think it would be fair to have the owners pack up their things and continue to do what they were doing if there was a chance that we were not going to close on the house. So, I told the real estate agent to tell *The Coffins* that there was a chance that we may not be able to close on the house; ironically, the owners of the Milo home were Sue and Joe Coffin. I never spoke to the agent again because Eddie died a month before our closing date.

TICKETS

After Eddie was put on life support and the tap was placed, he was moved up to the ICU; at first he was not responsive but he was stable. Eddie lay on a hospital bed surrounded by several IV bags filled with antibiotics to fight whatever illness he was afflicted with. When he was settled into his room and I saw that he was stable, I decided to take a breather; I went to the help desk on his floor and I asked to talk to a clergy person; I probably asked for a coffee too.

Naomi was waiting in the family area with Serena. She was trying to keep Serena calm and happy. The clergyperson was intended to do the same, for all of us. So, in honor of my request, a clergy person was found. I was introduced to a very sweet young woman; I was in a very bad place emotionally, so it was comforting that she had a genuinely warm disposition.

I can remember sitting in a room talking to her with Naomi and Serena sitting right beside me. We talked a little bit about Eddie's situation and I also expressed that I was feeling so guilty for the fact that the Disney trip was ruined for my baby; I thought the entire trip was over, that the tickets were a waste of The Dream Foundation's money.

Me being me, I exchanged some of my negative emotion for some positive emotion. I asked the clergy woman if she had any children and she told me she had a baby girl. I asked her if she had ever been to Disney; figured she had because she lived in those parts. She said she had but it was a goal to get back there again when she had the money. Well, I liked her, so I gave her two tickets to share with her little girl, someday. She was very happy, and it made me feel a little better too.

That same day, I gave my best friend a couple of tickets so she could take Serena to Disney the following day. But I had no idea that after I would finish talking with the clergy lady that my cousin Elaine would show up at the hospital; so it was a good thing that I didn't get *all manic* and start giving the tickets away to everyone. I had quite a few; enough for three people to go to Disney for three days.

I couldn't believe my eyes when I saw my cousin Elaine walking towards me in the hospital's family area. She was visiting Disney with her kids! I was amazed at the odds of finding a very close family member at such a time. I hadn't talked to her in about two years; it was an absolute miracle! She heard it through the family "grape vine" that I was in Florida with Eddie and Serena.

I was so blessed that on the very day that this tragedy occurred, God provided me with a support group. And they were with me on the night that Eddie was moved from the ER to the ICU. They shared in witnessing, for a brief time, Eddie being responsive. Eddie could hear my voice and he was moving his foot in response to my questions; Naomi and Elaine watched as Eddie squeezed my hand. He was aware of where he was, at that moment. But the next day, there was no response at all, and there would be none, for more than a week.

Soon it became Elaine's "duty" to help *me* ensure that Serena had some fun at Disney. I passed the torch to her, and it wasn't easy for me because I am used to having my baby with me wherever I go. I gave Elaine all the tickets that I had and I asked her to watch over my baby.

Serena was able to go to Disney with Elaine and her two kids. She spent three days in Disney; she got the full spread of Disney, as I stayed behind assisting with her father's care. If it hadn't been for Naomi and Elaine, Serena would have been robbed of the chance to see Disney.

When Elaine's vacation was ready to come to an end; she offered to take Serena back home with her to Maryland. She was going to watch over my baby and protect her. The hospital had strict rules about children being at the ICU. Besides, it was best for Serena to get away from all of the madness. She wanted to stay but she wanted to retire from her care giving duties even more; she helped me take care of her father for months while we were back home in Connecticut.

Eddie was still in a coma like state when Serena said good-bye to him. I remember she was supposed to wear a mask and not stay too long. I picked her up and put her face close to his and she kissed him and said "I love you Daddy, I hope you feel better". I put her down and she grabbed my hand and said, "Ok Mommy, I'm ready to go now." She was just excited about the fact that she was going on a journey to Maryland and that she was going to be with two of her cousins. She gathered up all of the souvenirs that I had bought her on the first day, and packed up the toys her Aunty Naomi bought her. She was ready to go so I walked outside with her down to Elaine's car. I helped her get in and I buckled her safely in her seat, then I kissed and hugged her goodbye. It was just another one of those painful life moments.

MEDICAL MARIJUANA

Ed had a lot of pain in his head so he required a heavy duty medication. The ventricular tap was very painful so the entire time he was at "Celebrity" Hospital he was on morphine.

Morphine was the strongest thing that they could give him for pain but when I asked Eddie if he was still feeling pain he signed with his hand yes, then I asked him if he wanted some "smoke" (marijuana) because when he was at home it was his drug of choice.

Ed always told his doctor that the weed made him feel less dizzy and he was able to have an appetite, plus it helped him to relax. Marijuana was something that Ed really liked all aspects of, so when he showed interest in medical marijuana, as his advocate and wife, I started to ask the nurses about it; I recommended that they provide him with some "creature comforts". I figured there couldn't be anything worse than the morphine that was running through his severely weakened veins; I figured the Delta 9 would be harmless.

Some nurses would laugh about my inquiries and others would just seem to ignore them. But after a couple of days I talked to a nurse who told me that there was a way to get THC for patients through their very own hospital pharmacy. She said all we needed to do was talk to an anesthesiologist.

It took a couple of days for the anesthesiologist to come to Ed's room. When he finally walked into the room I noticed he was short, his hair was messy, he was wearing glasses and his shirt was half tucked in and his collar was flipped up. Obviously, the man had a little bit of freedom to be on the wild side. He probably took on a much more laid back disposition compared to his colleagues. After all, he was the "drug guy"

He loudly said "Mr. Haney!" Ed's eyes got wide because it was a new voice and one full of energy. He asked Ed, "would you like some marijuana?" Ed shook his head yes a couple of times. Then the doctor said, "You got it buddy, I'm going to write you out a script."

The next thing we knew, a nurse came walking into Ed's room carrying, cocktail waitress style, a tray with a little cup containing some liquid.

"I have your treat Mr. Haney." She seemed as excited as a school girl to be able to present this "treat" to Ed; of course he was very happy about the delivery. So, with a shit eat'n grin on her face, she put it through his feeding tube.

Every 4 hours he started receiving his doses of morphine and marijuana; the prescribed marijuana was meant to help Eddie with his pain and discomfort and it was meant to settle his fried nerves.

It was great that he got that because it made him happy. As his friend, first and foremost, I always went out of my way to make him happy and "hook" him up but others would persecute him for smoking marijuana; for years people put him down over his marijuana use. Even in his last year of his life and knowing that it made him feel better—they would still criticize him for "indulging".

In my mind, people who smoke marijuana should not feel guilty, especially if they are sick and using it for medicinal purposes!

THE SUFFERING

Now, I realize that we are only human; mankind makes mistakes and accidents happen. But in some places human error is less forgivable; that's why I must tell of the care my husband received while he was a patient at "Celebrity" Hospital. This explanation of care is **not meant to bash or discredit "Celebrity" Hospital**, instead please try to view it as a tool to help stop it from happening anymore.

As time has gone by I have come to realize that I am only harboring the guilt and pain from my experience with Eddie's passing.

I am haunted by the outcome of his cancer battle. I have been left behind to a world of guilt and overwhelming sadness. But I know in my heart that I can and will over come the suffering that I am left with. Through this book and this very chapter, I can expel all that is consuming my heart; to start, I must tell of the medical care Eddie received while he was a patient at "Celebrity" Hospital

I contacted **"Celebrity's"** Risk Management and I did get a response; my goal for contacting Risk Management was to make the staff at **"Celebrity"** Hospital understand where they so terribly went wrong with my husband's care; I relayed to the Risk Management team that I was concerned for the welfare of other patients as well. And I made it clear that I was not satisfied with some levels of care which were provided to my husband; I have made it a personal obligation of mine to inform others of the risks involving mouth care and other medical procedures and I am confident that what I have seen and learned from my husband's suffering will help others who are faced with the same type of situation he was faced with.

It is so important to play the role of advocate for the ones we love because we are their best hope for survival and proper medical care.

Wives, caregivers, and family advocates are like gold to a patient.

But what if perhaps I did the opposite for my husband. Maybe I truly did him an injustice when I allowed doctors to interrupt his death? He would have died if they hadn't placed that tube down his throat and he would have died if they hadn't drained the fluid from his head; he just simply would have died on April 9, 2007 if I hadn't allowed for his death to be interrupted; he should have died on that day, technically that is.

If I didn't opt for the life support and if perhaps Serena and I had returned back from the Magic Kingdom just an hour or two later, he would have died peacefully in his king size bed with the impression that his wish for Serena was being fulfilled; but I just couldn't let him go and now I'm suffering with guilt.

On the night that Eddie was brought to the ER, I couldn't resist, I had to try to save him; he had four of the most beautiful children to live for.

Well, I did play hero to my man by putting him on life support; I woke him up and brought him back to par and he was even coming home; he really was. But it was my own selfish love for him that caused me to interrupt his death. I'm the one to blame for any of his suffering; granted I didn't do the physical part, like gouging a hole in his mouth and destroying his lips or causing him any pain; still, I did act as the tool to let the neglect come right in.

The guilt that surrounds the interruption has caused me to have to deal with PTSD (Post Traumatic Stress Disorder). I get flashbacks and sometimes it is hard to focus on anything but dwelling over Eddie. I often imagine myself laying with him in his coffin with my head on his chest; resting in peace together. I have really tapped into my dark side over the past couple of years since his death. I'm obsessed in some ways to keep his memory alive, hence this book, and I am so consumed with sorrow on a daily basis.

What I saw him go through and what he had to endure was truly something on a biblical level. Actually, I remember reading about Job in the Bible while I was with Eddie at the hospital; I read it to him and I told him he reminded me of Job.

Some of the suffering that he went through was nothing like most cancer patients go through. All the blood and all the pain, not related to cancer, were horrible to see; it was as though he was afflicted, like Job, with every kind of pain.

Eddie was in a position where he couldn't communicate verbally because of the stroke and he was paralyzed on his left side; plus his right arm was tied down for the most part; I know he was pissed off at the fact that he felt like prisoner in his own bed.

Now, looking back, I'm sure that if Eddie could have spoken, he would have threatened to hurt anyone who touched his mouth again! And he would have started first with the nurse who was suctioning out the spit from his throat.

Each time a nurse would suction the spit from his mouth; it apparently hurt him because he punched me in my thigh three times. And he really hit me hard, to the point I cried because I was physically hurt, but at the same time I was emotionally torn because I knew something was wrong and he was hurting; a nurse even said "Mr. Haney, you can't hit your wife!" She meant no harm, I believe she wasn't intentionally trying to hurt my husband, but even so, she was; they all were.

The true nightmare of it all, to me, is that I was helping them hurt him. I was holding his arm down to stop him from grabbing the suction tube. I stopped him, I pinned him; just so that the nurses could do their job.

But it came to the point that I couldn't bare to see him fight off the nurses any longer; I knew something was seriously wrong but he couldn't put it into words. When I asked him if it hurt, he shook his head to say yes.

I felt so bad because I couldn't understand why it was hurting him so badly, just getting suctioned; I began to explore his mouth to see if I could find out why he was in pain. No nurse ever looked deep into his mouth and no nurse examined his mouth in anyway; it wasn't until I demanded that closer attention be made to his mouth.

I borrowed a nurse's flash light and I started to carefully pry open his mouth with my fingers. His mouth was bloody and extremely dry; he could no longer swallow on his own, one of the problems with a brainstem tumor; among other critical non voluntary functions. The life support tube was still in his mouth when I started to explore it with the light, so there wasn't much space in his mouth; the tube took up much of it.

His mouth barely opened at all; it was all bloody inside and thrush had taken over his tongue. The thrush was yellowish brown and it looked like mold spots all over his tongue. It looked so bad that I can remember asking the nurse "is that dead man's mouth?" To me, it looked like death.

But once I pointed out the thrush to a nurse, she got the approval to start treating it with a Nystatin, a polyene antifungal drug.

About a week after Ed had started being treated for his thrush; he was taken off of life support. Up till the day that he was taken off the life support, he was suctioned on a regular basis and he still complained of extreme pain. It wasn't until the tubes were out that I could get a real good look in Eddie's mouth.

Even without the tubes it was extremely difficult for Ed's mouth to open. When I was able to get a good view up into the roof of his mouth I was shocked at what I found. I could see that there was a hole in his hard pallet. It was a bloody mess in his mouth and now I knew where all the blood was coming from.

The suction tubes were a slightly hard plastic; every time the nurses would go in and suction the spit that he wasn't able to swallow, from his throat, the nurses hit the roof of his mouth with the hard plastic tube; they barely made it to the back of his throat.

If you really think about it, imagine the tube in your mouth and you bite down slightly and try to put something else in there, just see how far it gets before it hits the roof of your mouth. And imagine being a patient laying there who can't say "that's hitting the roof of my mouth" or think of a person who is in a coma like state, who can't communicate at all, not even with their eyes!

He had so much blood in his mouth; it started to clump up on his tongue but none of the nurses were seeing what I was seeing because they weren't really listening to me and they weren't looking. And I was so upset to see his mouth in that condition, and I couldn't understand how the nurses let this happen to him.

No nurse looked in his mouth; not until I threatened someone to do it—when I say threatened I mean—don't fuck with my man or I will kick your ass, kind of attitude; always does the trick!

The blood that covered his tongue dried up into clots. The blood clots were so bad that when I attempted to help him peel them off, just to clean his mouth, it literally would rip a hole into his tongue like a crater. The blood had dried onto his tongue; it was like school glue that had dried up, so when I tried to pull the clot off, he started to bleed. I never wanted to hurt him so I stopped trying to remove the clots.

I was confused as to how he got this way. How could the nurses be so unaware of what was going on in his mouth? I always heard that mouth care was among the most critical areas of care for a patient.

In addition to the concern I had over the hole that the suction tubes left, I was worried about the tape that was on his face. It was around the mouth piece of the life support tubes. What was worrying me was that the tape was changed only one time, and only when I requested it after only a few days following the first time he was incubated. But the second time the tape was removed wasn't until he was taken off of the life support several days later.

Before he was taken off of the life support I asked his nurses to please change the tape again. I asked for about three days but it was never done; the tape was starting to get thin. Instead it being the normal tape shape, the rectangle shape, it was starting to become more like a string. It was getting stringy because the tape was wearing. And it started to press in to his lip in such a way that it was creasing his lip, sinking into his lip and gradually compressing into his lip causing a valley in his lip; the tape was cutting into him.

Even though it was plain to see and I made several requests for the tape to be changed, it went undone and Eddie was ultimately wounded, induced by staff. I can remember a couple of nurses and a respiratory tech telling me not to worry because soon he would be taken off life support and the tape could wait till then.

When it finally came time for the respiratory techs to remove all the tape and life support I was very apprehensive about leaving the room. The respiratory tech told me he wanted me to leave the room so that he could do what was needed to remove the tubes.

Well, I strongly informed him that Eddie's lips were sensitive. I told him I was concerned that if he ripped the tape off too quickly he would make Eddie bleed and hurt him. Eddie's lips were not bloody and they were completely intact, with the exception of the valley in his lips. The only blood he had on him was from the hole in the roof of his mouth.

I went against my better judgment and I waited outside the door while they took the tubes out. I waited for days and days for my husband to be freed from the breathing machine. I was so excited that it was coming out; I just wanted them to get it over with and get him breathing on his own again. So I didn't stand in their way.

Shockingly, when the tech called me into the room after they removed everything, I looked at my husband. He had no lips left on his face! When the tech ripped the tape off, they ripped his lips off with it! Where his lips had been, there was nothing but blood.

The blood was the consistency of a bloody nose. The skin that made his lips was totally removed. So there I was, looking at my poor husband's mouth. He looked liked a dead man with clots and yeast on his tongue and a hole on the roof of his mouth, with no lips.

So let's see, he came into the hospital with no open wounds, no blood and signs of trauma but after days in the care of "Celebrity" he became a damaged man. His mouth was torn up, his lips were gone and he was being treated for who knows what; when Eddie was brought to the ER I told the neurologist that Eddie had, what I thought was, an ear infection.

The neurologist was "pretty sure" it was meningitis; I disagreed. It took several days for me to convince the infectious disease doctor to allow Eddie to be seen by an ENT. And of course as my intuition would have it, when the ENT viewed Eddie's ears he found an infection and severe swimmer ear. The next day Eddie had tubes placed in his ears and after the surgery the ENT prescribed cipro, specific for the ear, in the dropper form.

Within the next day Eddie started coming out of his coma like state; I always said, "When we have the flu or cold or even a terrible ear infection, we generally have a fever with body aches and all we want to do is sleep".

I think that is what was happening with Eddie, he feels like shit, so he's staying asleep. That was my view on it; I still think it was right.

Granted, he did have a stroke, which knocked him down pretty hard, but that coupled with a very bad flu / ear infection would definitely take its toll on any person.

When he did come out of his stupor I tended to his care for the majority of the day. During the countless number of hours that I spent lovingly tending to my husband's every need; I would nurse and help to heal his wounded lips and care for his assaulted mouth with salt packets left over from my lunches; the salt water on his tongue was the only thing that removed the blood clots from his tongue without causing a bloody crater.

Sometimes I would put eye drops in his eyes; Eddie suffered from dry eyes for several years and he used eye drops to help alleviate his dry eyes. As his wife, I was the only one who knew about his dry eyes so I thought it was odd when a nurse asked me "did you give him his eye drops today?" Surprised that she knew, I said "yes".

I began to notice that when his hand was free he would lift it up and rub his right eye; he rubbed it like a tired person would when they first get up.

Sometimes I would pull his hand down because I was afraid that he would yank a tube out of his head or nose.

I wasn't sure why he was rubbing it so frequently; I soon found out. A couple of days later I noticed a nurse who was about to put cipro in Eddie's eye! Suddenly I realized why his eye was looking so blood shot and why he was rubbing it; some of the nurses were placing the cipro ear drops in his eye, instead. My God, he was in so much pain; his eye was on fire.

A nurse by the name of Judy, she was an excellent nurse, told me, "Mrs. Haney, I'm so sorry but you were right, cipro has been used in his eye." I don't know if she ever made a report of it, and who knows if the one I made to Risk Management was taken seriously. All I know is it was true and it was admitted; these truths are valuable because they are evidence and confirmation that real risks do exist in the medical world, and people need to be protected by careless and incompetent medical staff. I'm sure there are many people who are suffering at the hands of another right at this moment.

A BLOODY KISS GOOD-BYE

He was in room 302 of the ICU. From his bed he could see the double doors which led out to the corridor leaving the ICU; his room was the last room on that end of the ward.

I trusted no one with his care; it worried me fiercely just the thought of leaving him for a few hours. As his advocate I spoke for him and I protected him, so leaving him, again, was the most horrendous event to ever take place in my life. He hated that fact that I was leaving and I could tell he was deeply saddened by the fact that "this was it" this was goodbye.

I worked so hard to keep Eddie alive because I wanted nothing more than for him to live! He needed to get back to Connecticut so his children could be with him but I was so worried that he would die in Florida and I would have to bury him there. All I could think of was his family and friends, I didn't want to rob them of the chance to be present at his funeral and I wanted him buried close to home in the VA cemetery as we had arranged.

We had discussed the whole trip back to Connecticut. He was going to fly home on a medical flight and I was going to drive our car back home and pick Serena up along the way. Together she and I were going to meet Eddie off the plane in Connecticut. I was working myself up for a couple of days; there was no way in hell that I wanted to leave him.

When it came time for me to leave I walked over to my husband and I told him that I was going to meet him off of the medical plane in Connecticut in less than 24 hours; he was due to fly out, on April 27, 2007. And instantly, after I told Eddie that it was time to go, he put up his right hand and with his pointer finger he pointed up to the sky to say wait! Oh my God, I was so crushed inside as I walked over to him and got as close as I could; he reached out for me and he softly grabbed my cheeks, looked deeply into my eyes and pulled my head down to his chest and laid my head to his heart. I was crying and bleeding inside and all that I truly wanted was to stay with him, but I couldn't . . . . my heart told me it was time to get Serena.

Painfully, after a few minutes I lifted my head and I expressed to him the most intimate words I had ever shared with him; it was a moment that only a man and wife could share, so deeply personal and painful.

I hadn't kissed Eddie on the lips the whole time we were in the hospital. His lips and mouth were not kissable for the most part. He either had a tube in his mouth or major damage to his lips and mouth. It wasn't until the day I was saying good-bye that I kissed him.

I looked into his eyes and I gently lifted the back of his head, as if I were filling my hands with water. Then, when we were face to face, I kissed his lips. I pressed down firmly so he could really feel my love. After I kissed him he had a look of excitement and amazement because, like I said we hadn't kissed in eighteen days; I knew he was happy about kissing me. I said "Eddie did you like that?" He shook his head yes and he smiled with his wide eyes; I kissed his lips again, then I kissed his forehead. Heartbreakingly, I left behind a bloody kiss print; the blood from his lips, were covering mine.

There were tears, as heavy as the biggest rain drop, rolling down my face while I told him good-bye. But before I actually walked out of his room, and with so much regret, in my very soul, I told him that he could stop fighting and holding on for my sake. I told him I couldn't stand to see him suffer. With tears **pouring** down my face I turned around and I walked out of his room; *I swear that my heart was cut in half when I left that hospital.*

I drove for fifteen hours; along the way I stopped at a pay phone somewhere in Georgia and I called Eddie's nurse. I wanted to know his status and she assured me he was doing well. I told her to tell him I loved him and that I would see him soon. I also told her to let him know I was in Georgia and still heading north up Interstate 95.

Finally, I made it to Maryland where Serena laid sound asleep at my cousin's house. It was around 3 am. I walked into the room Serena was in.

I scooped her up in my arms while she still slept. I just needed to hold my baby. The only reason I left Eddie was to get our baby so that she could be there in Connecticut after he got off the plane.

I didn't want to fly with Eddie and leave my car behind in Florida because there would be no way to retrieve Serena. I held her so tight; she was so soft and precious to me and the only person who could truly feel my pain. After a few minutes with Serena, I laid her back down and went into the kitchen and called "Celebrity" Hospital.

It was very early in the morning when I asked to speak to the nurse on duty. She told me that Ed was critical and he had been placed back on life support! I was shocked because I had only been away from him for fifteen hours and already he was back on life support! It was insane to me, I had worked for eighteen days helping him recover at the hospital and when I left him he was off of life support.

When I left he had no tubes in his head, no problems except his weakness and paralysis from his stroke. The tumor was still a major risk but I was hoping to get Eddie back to Connecticut for more chemotherapy treatments. His flu was gone, his kidneys were functioning well and he was fully aware.

The nurse put the surgeon on the line and he asked me if he could have permission to put the ventricular tap back into his head because he had fears that Ed had more fluid building up. I said "no"! I didn't want anyone else to touch him! He told me it would likely kill him anyway if he redid the same procedure he had just done only eighteen days earlier in the ER.

The doctor told me that I needed to get back there ASAP, but I was dead tired from driving all night and I would have never made it to him on time if I drove! I was afraid that Serena would be at risk in the car with me because of my lethargy.

To make matters worse, the doctor gave the phone to a nurse to speak with me; I can recall arguing with her; she was a southern woman with an annoying Southern accent and she constantly referred to me as Sugar, Honey, Sweetie and whatever. I told her that I needed her to treat me like a grown woman and stop patronizing me.

I was delegating the type of care to provide my husband with but she kept insisting that I was making the wrong choices; I was telling her to do whatever she could to keep him alive, I told her I was on my way and that I needed her to keep him alive! But like I said, she continued to patronize me with her honey pies and sugar peas! What an ignorant person she was; I hated her. I remember she even said at one point, "he's gone . . . . no he's back." She drove me crazy to talk to but she was the only one who I could talk to about what was happening to Eddie; I was in Maryland and he was in Florida.

The only other person that I had to talk to from Florida was Leah. She was a Jehovah's Witness whom I had befriended. A beautiful and close friend of mine, Brie, called her from back home in CT and coordinated a meeting between us. Leah showed up at the hospital on the very night that Eddie was taken from the hotel by the ambulance.

And it was her that I called when I was in Maryland; she was already at Eddie's room when I called her. The hospital recognized that Leah and I had become close during the eighteen days at the ICU, so they felt comfortable answering her questions about Eddie. But when it came time for them to allow her at his bedside while I was stuck in Maryland, the nursing staff did not permit it. Not until I demanded it, that is.

I can remember screaming at the nurses, warning them that if they didn't let my spiritual friends near his body, I would sue them for not respecting my wishes. I told the nurses that I didn't want him to die alone. One nurse, the southern one, said, "He is with us now, he won't die alone." It made me ill to think he was all alone with them; after all they were the ones I had trusted to take care of him in the first place.

While I was on the phone with Leah, after the nurses finally let her be in the room to observe what was taking place, she told me what was happening to Eddie. She said the nurses were busily working on keeping his heart rate managed. I was asking her to explain to me in detail what was happening; I told her to give messages to the nurse for me, and she did.

One was "Stop that NOW!" I was referring to the moment when Leah told me the nurses were busy doing mouth care! They told Leah that she couldn't put the phone to Eddie's ear for me to speak to him; the reason was due to that retched mouth care again; Leah told me that in the midst of all the "heart rate trauma and breathing difficulty", Eddie was putting his hand up to push the nurses away from his bloody mouth; they were obviously STILL hurting my man. So, there he was, "dying", as the nurses put it, and they were still performing mouth care. I just don't get it to this day; I was so emotionally distraught.

My cousin Elaine interrupted my conversation with Leah and she told me that my uncle Robert had many frequent flyer miles from all of his business trips; I called him early that morning and I told him about my crisis and he simply asked me exactly what I needed from him.

I told him I needed to fly me and my baby BACK to Florida to be with Eddie before he died! And about 10 minutes later, he had purchased and arranged for Serena and me to catch a round trip flight out of Baltimore only 30 minutes later.

I grabbed Serena's hand and told her she needed to be brave one more time. At first she was scared about the idea of flying but I gingerly explained to Serena that there was nothing scarier than what her dad was going through, and then she agreed and packed up her things. Elaine brought us to the airport and we boarded the plane and headed to Chicago, yeah Chicago.

It made no sense but we had to go up to Chicago to change planes then head back down to Florida. It was absolute torture for me to head into the opposite direction of my dying husband.

My only sense of comfort was that I had my baby next to me. We were about to find out Ed's fate together. One of my fears was that I would have to return back to Serena bearing news of her daddy's death. I dreaded that thought so to me it was a miracle that she was with me. The flight to Chicago took us an hour or so and it was within that hour that Eddie died.

When the plane finally landed, I just wanted to push my way through the crowd but instead I waited my turn. I was nearly delirious with fatigue but I had to hurry and get off the plane to get to my husband. Our new friends Steve and Nancy were waiting for us as we walked to the end of the plane tunnel into the airport; they were also Jehovah's Witnesses. We were back in sunny Florida only to experience extreme darkness.

Steve drove while Serena and I impatiently sat in the back seat of his car. We were extremely anxious to get to Eddie. I borrowed Steve's phone and I called "Celebrity" Hospital. When the southern nurse picked up the phone she told me he was dead. I couldn't believe it and neither could Serena!

The medical staff at "Celebrity" was expecting Serena and me to come view his body. So when we arrived they met us in the family waiting room to talk to us about Ed's passing. A clergyman walked us to outside Ed's room.

When we first saw him his eyes were wide open and yellowed. He looked like he had really been through hell. All of the tubes were still hanging out of his body. He had a catheter in his heart, a life support tube hanging from his mouth only half assembled and he was left uncovered. It was no way to present a body for a now widow and orphan. I was disgusted and I was in shock. I couldn't cry. Serena didn't cry either. Together we were in shock. The last thing that I can remember the supervising nurse saying to me was, **"he died because you left him; you were apparently his life force."**

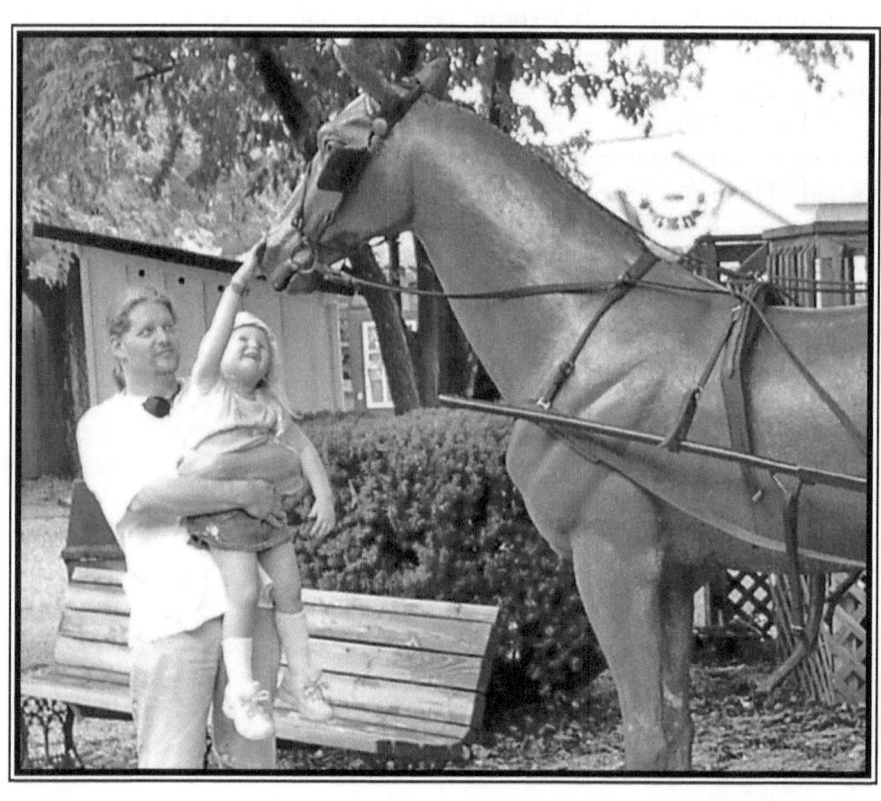

www.ingramcontent.com/pod-product-compliance
Lightning Source LLC
Chambersburg PA
CBHW050340290526
45785CB00006B/2566